The Last

Hurrah

A Living Workbook for a Happy Ending

Mary Ann Burrows

Natural Narrative Publishing

Copyright 2023 Mary Ann Burrows
Edited by Jess Lomas

All rights reserved. No part of this publication may be reproduced, distributed, or transmitted in any form or by any means, including photocopying, recording or other electronic or mechanical methods, without the prior written permission of the publisher, except in the case of brief quotations embodied in critical reviews and certain other noncommercial uses permitted by copyright law. For permission requests and author inquiries: maryannb@eastlink.ca

Maryannburrows.com

I dedicate this book to

Malia Johnson,
the 90-year-old woman
that I met at Starbucks
in Kihei, Maui, Hawaii
who generously shared with me
her very elaborate 'Last Hurrah' plan,
sparking the idea for this book.

The Last Hurrah: A Living Workbook," is intended for informational and educational purposes only. While every effort has been made to ensure the accuracy and relevance of the content, the author and publisher make no representations or warranties regarding the completeness, accuracy, or applicability of the information provided.

This book does not constitute legal, financial, medical, or professional advice of any kind. It is not a substitute for consulting with qualified professionals such as lawyers, health professionals, or financial advisors. The author and publisher disclaim any liability, loss, or risk incurred as a direct or indirect consequence of using or applying any information presented in book.

Contents

Preface	7
Introduction	13
1. Reflecting on Your Life	17
2. Envisioning Your Last Hurrah	37
My Dream Big First Draft	
3. You Get the Last Word	47
My Self Authored Obituary	
4. The Guest List	63
5. Crafting the Program	77
My Self- Authored Eulogy	
My Last Hurrah Plan Details	
6. Writing Your Farewell Message	107
My Personal Notes/Private Letters	
7. The Practicalities of Parting	121
Making Things Easier for Loved Ones	
Where my documents are located	
Who to contact	
Keys, Codes and Access	
8. Care and Resting Place Preferences	137
Helpful Terms	
End of Life Care	
My Burial Plan	
Epitaphs, Ashes,	
My Final Outfit	
9. The Final Chapter	175
My Ethical Will	
Epilogue	185
Acknowledgements	187
Resources	191
Directory for My Loved Ones	195

Preface

I really don't want to talk about dying. I love living. Nevertheless, here we are having the conversation that most people dread. The death talk. Most people are afraid to talk about death, as if the mere act of discussing it might summon its unwelcome presence. This misconception is leaving people unprepared for the inevitable. We are all going to eventually die. We need to talk about our ending.

By pure happenstance, this book came to life after a random chat with a woman named Malia Johnson at Starbucks. Malia is a nonagenarian living on the beautiful island of Maui, Hawaii. She's vibrant, witty, and brimming with stories, her life a rich tapestry of academic achievements, a fulfilling career, and adventures in both love and life.

What truly captivated me was Malia's colourful life history and her progressive outlook towards the end of her life. Despite being 90 years old and still dancing and driving, she was a huge football fan and in pretty good health. She wasn't anticipating her passing any time soon, yet she was also eager to discuss her earthly departure with me. Remarkably, she even whipped out a detailed, typed plan she had personally crafted for her "Celebration of Life Party." Her plan meticulously outlined every aspect, from the chosen musicians, complete with their contact details, to a carefully curated playlist and guest list for the event. Her plan was a powerful declaration of her life and choices, wisely premeditated by herself as her "last hurrah," a celebration of herself for after she was gone that showcased who she was and how she had lived for 90 years on Earth.

Meeting Malia led me to reflect on my own family: What were my aging parents' wishes? I had no idea. My daughter had been asking me for years about my final plans, but I hadn't communicated my wishes to anyone. Why was talking about death so daunting?

The necessity of writing this book became clear. I came to understand how vital it is to have a conversation about our death with the people we love. I wanted to write a book so that I could talk about the inevitable with my parents and make losing me more manageable for my children.

This book is a living workbook, meaning that it serves as a dynamic and ever-changing document that encourages your ongoing updates and additions, empowering you, as it's author, to contribute to it continuously until you feel that you have completed your journey.

This constant evolution ensures that the workbook remains relevant, effective, and aligned with you, your thoughts, needs and aspirations throughout your experience with it.

Meeting Malia made me realize that my purpose extends beyond simply living a life worthy of celebration. It includes the responsibility to thoughtfully plan that ultimate celebration of departure, ensuring it truly reflects the richness and uniqueness of life.

Here's to my wild and untamed dreams,

of belly laughs by sunlit streams,

to every tear, to every scar,

Welcome to my Last Hurrah!

Introduction

The Last Hurrah was designed to help all of us have the difficult death conversation. Although, careful preparation is no match for the unpredictability of death; most of us don't get to choose our time. The process of articulating your final wishes in this book empowers both you and your loved ones. This book offers a structured yet flexible and somewhat joyful approach to end-of-life planning. The goal of this book is to transform end-of-life planning from a daunting task into an opportunity for reflection and celebration. This book is an invaluable resource for individuals at any stage of life and a thoughtful tool for those wanting to have these conversations with their aging parents.

Through this workbook, you'll find ways to thoughtfully engage with and shape the narrative of your life's end. It's not just about planning; it's about rediscovering and reaffirming the vibrancy of your life and ensuring your story is known so you can be celebrated in a way that is commemorative, not somber.

By writing down your story, you get to craft an ending as unique as your journey, allowing the last chapter of your life to end with a 'big hurrah'—a true reflection of a well-lived life.

Your journey through this workbook begins with a reflective expedition, inviting you to explore the depths of your personal story, including a glimpse into your history and achievements. This introspective start paves the way for "Envisioning Your Last Hurrah," a chapter that encourages you to dream without limits. This imaginative exercise is not only fun but also reveals aspects of yourself that you might have overlooked, helping you incorporate these elements into your ultimate celebration.

Next, the workbook guides you in "You Get the Last Word." Here, you are in control, holding the pen that writes the concluding chapter of your life. This empowering section gives you the authority to decide everything from who will attend your final gathering to the design of the farewell ceremony and even crafting your own obituary.

Following these imaginative and creative explorations, the workbook focuses on the practicalities of parting. I'll lead you through the logistics of your departure, including outlining your care preferences and selecting a resting place. This ensures that all your wishes are well-thought-out and clearly communicated.

The Last Hurrah provides a straightforward approach to essential end-of-life considerations, from the whereabouts of your Will to the fate of your social media accounts. It covers everything from your preferred final send-off details to the legacy you wish to leave behind, ensuring nothing is overlooked. This is a living workbook to update throughout life, ensuring your final chapter is as well-planned as the life you've led, giving you and your loved ones peace of mind.

"Looking back at my life's voyage, I can only say that it has been a golden trip."

Ginger Rogers

-1-
Reflecting on Your Life

Let's begin by taking a stroll down memory lane, picking out the bits of your life that made you laugh, cry, and jump for joy. It's like mapping out a final, grand adventure where you get to sprinkle in a bit of everything you've loved, learned, and lived for. Think about the people who've been your cheerleaders, the places that felt like home, and the dreams you've danced with. Your final chapter is not just about tying up loose ends but more about gathering everything together and then throwing one last party that's all about you—a celebration of every high, low, and crazy twist your life's story has taken.

Think of this space as your life journal. A place for you to document the myriad experiences, people, and events that have shaped who you are. Writing about yourself and your life can bring up a lot of feelings. Expect to feel happy and sad, angry, and regretful and also expect to feel a lot of joy. Remember, these feelings are all normal because writing your story out is not only an act of reminiscence but a journey of appreciation and acknowledgement of your precious life. From the details of your birthdate to the intricate web of your achievements, your relationships, and beliefs, each aspect you jot down is a crucial part of your story. This is your life.

So, lets start at YOUR beautiful beginning…

Writing Exercise: *Grab a pencil and settle into a comfortable chair with a cup of hot tea or coffee and let's write. Over the next few pages, you'll have the opportunity to write the outline of your life with the details that are specific to you, such as your birth date, the places you've called home, your earliest family memories and some important milestones.*

My Life In My Words

Your story started on the day you were born. Your story is unique to you and it's important to share it. Sharing your story helps people feel closer to you in the present and gives them something to hold onto for generations to come.

My given name(s): _____

Place of birth: _____

Date of birth: _____

My parents or those who raised me:

_____

My siblings

_____

A few childhood memories:

Schools I attended, courses I completed.

Key moments and achievements:

Marriage(s) and children:

Significant life events:

Interesting things about me:

The values and beliefs that define me (things that give me a sense of meaning, value, and purpose):

A few things that I survived:

How the world has changed in my lifetime:

My hobbies:

My favourite poem:

The one book that changed my life:

My favourite songs:

My bucket list of things I have yet to do:

A special story about my life:

When I was younger, I wish I had known:

Something that I want to be remembered for: (my legacy)

_____

_____

_____

Above everything else I want my family to know this about me and my life:

_____

_____

_____

Sum your legacy up into one sentence:

_____

Tracing Your Roots Building a Family Tree

Additional Project: *Create a family tree. A visual record of your ancestry shows how the people in your life fit together. Use the family tree template in Microsoft Excel to get started or use a Family Tree app. Reach out to your relatives to get started.*

As you gather information, reach out to your relatives. Ask them for names, birthdates and places of birth of your aunts and uncles, your cousins. This process is a beautiful opportunity for connection, sparking conversations and uncovering stories that might have been forgotten. Each name, date, and place you add to your tree revives a piece of history, offering insights into your heritage and strengthening family bonds

Use the following pages to write down what you can remember about your family tree, such as the names of your grandparents and where they were born. Write out as much information that you can remember and you will see that your tree will begin to grow. You can write it out on a separate piece of paper and slip this valuable record between these pages. Your family tree is not just a chart; it's a living, breathing chronicle of your family's journey through generations. Sharing this with your family members is a gift of knowledge and belonging. It's a legacy that will be cherished and, most importantly, preserved for future generations. Your family will thank you for taking the time to weave together these threads of the past, bringing clarity and a sense of unity to your shared heritage.

Two well-known sites that offer help with family trees or ancestry are:

Ancestry: https://www.ancestry.com

MyHeritage: https://www.myheritage.com

My Roots

Include the names, birth and death dates, places of birth and occupations of the following ancestors, (if known)

My maternal grandparents:

My paternal grandparents:

My maternal great-grandparents:

My paternal great-grandparents:

The names of other relatives in my family tree:

Important things I want to share about my family history:

Use a pencil to draw your family tree and fill it in.

"Everything you can imagine is real."

Pablo Picasso

-2-

Envisioning Your Last Hurrah

After reflecting on the rich narrative of your life's story and the intricate branches of your family tree, we now turn our gaze towards a celebration that encapsulates the essence of your amazing journey. Your Last Hurrah isn't just any party; it's a grand homage to the life you've lived, the challenges you've overcome, and the joy you've spread.

Imagine a gathering where every moment you cherished, every person who touched your heart, and every dream you pursued comes together like a resplendent love story. Imagine an event where each chapter of your life comes to life like scenes from an epic tale. As the architect of this grand celebration; you are its heart and soul, you are the reason for its existence.

You, my friend, are the guest of honour.

Before we get to the final party details, I want to first spend some time deep in the realms of your boundless imagination. You've had a life. You are alive right now and with that in mind, I invite you to use your imagination to dream up your ultimate celebration without the constraints of practicality.

Spend an afternoon or two picturing every tiny detail, from the joyous sounds of a huge marching band to the majestic ambiance of being paddled out to sea. Visualize who will be there, what melodies will fill the air, the flavours that will tantalize the taste buds of your guests and the theme that will flow through the air capturing the essence of your life's journey.

The following pages are your canvas to paint a vivid picture of your ideal farewell, a space where your dreams are given free rein. Don't hold back, ask yourself how you want to be celebrated.

How would it feel to arrive at the party of your life on the back of an elephant, (if so, write this down.) Do you want your ashes to be shot into the air from a cannon, (write that down, too.) As you delve into this creative exploration, remember this exercise is more than just fantasizing about an extravagant event; it's an intimate process of reflecting on your life's unique story and rediscovering what makes you tick.

In this celebration, every element, from the decor to the setting, tells a part of your story. If you've cherished nature, let there be elements of the outdoors, from floral arrangements that remind you of your favorite gardens to a sunset backdrop that mirrors your love for the twilight skies. If art has been your solace, let the space be adorned with representations of your favourite pieces, or better yet, your own creations. Are you a poet? Let your guests know.

This fusion of past, present, and future in your celebration does more than just mark the end of a journey. It's a confluence of all the moments that have shaped you, a kaleidoscope of your life's myriad facets. It's a vibrant testament, not just to the life you lived but to the enduring essence of your spirit that will continue to inspire and influence.

As we turn these next few pages, we are not just planning an event; we are crafting an enduring legacy. It's a legacy that captures the quintessence of your being, a celebration that transcends the conventional, embodying the uniqueness of your journey.

Imagining Your Ultimate Celebration

Think beyond your limits. Your final celebration might not feature you arriving on an elephant, but why not entertain the thought? This writing exercise is about weaving fantastical elements into the ultimate celebratory event.

Start by jotting down an unrestricted plan, focusing on your deepest desires and values. This is not only about planning an event; it's a journey into the heart of your legacy. Envision your ideal celebration without worrying about cost or time.

Engage Your Senses

Take a moment to reflect. Picture the essence of your ideal celebration, allowing it to come alive in your thoughts. In this moment of reflection, forget practicalities. Concentrate on your true self. Listen to what your heart says, and let these feelings guide your vision.

Visualize: Let your eyes paint the canvas of your life and legacy. What images spring forth? Think of colors, shapes, and scenes that embody your journey.

Listen: Tune into the soundtrack of your life. What songs resonate with your personality? Imagine the melodies and rhythms that define your character.

Savour with Taste: Recall the flavors that bring you joy. Which foods and drinks tantalize your taste buds and are synonymous with your happiest moments?

Embrace with Touch: Think of the textures and sensations that comfort you. Is it the softness of a well-loved book, the smoothness of a cherished piece of clothing, or the warmth of sunlight on your face?

Inhale with Smell: Breathe in deeply. What scents evoke memories and feelings? Is it the aroma of your favorite meal cooking, the fresh air of your beloved places, or a scent tied to a fond memory?

Reflect on Your Passions and Hobbies: What activities ignite your spirit? Consider how these interests paint a vivid picture of who you are.

Contemplate Unique Themes: Delve into aspects that uniquely define you – your favorite era, hobbies, fashion styles, and colors. How do these elements weave together to portray your personality?

Consider Favourite Places: Where does your heart feel most at home? Visualize a place that brings peace or exhilaration – a serene garden, the rhythmic ocean, a vibrant cityscape, or a tranquil forest.

Ponder Wishes, Hopes, and Dreams: What aspirations light up your heart? Let your deepest desires and dreams come to the forefront, shaping a vision of your future that's rich in personal fulfillment.

As you explore these sensory dimensions, let them guide your insights. When you're ready, capture these thoughts on paper, weaving them into a tapestry that uniquely represents YOU.

Writing Exercise: Grab a pen and write out the party of your wildest dreams. Without limits, cost constraints, or location restrictions. This initial draft is your chance to let your imagination run wild, and some of these ideas will find their way into your ultimate party plan.

My No-Limits Wild Celebration Dream First Draft

-3-

You Get the Last Word: Writing Your Obituary

Yes, you can write your own obituary. What an honor it is to be able to choose what people will read about you after you are gone. Plus, you get to pick out your own photo. Why leave this for others to decide?

I have left two blank pages here for you to make notes. Or, if you prefer, slide a printed copy of your obituary along with your favorite photograph or yourself in between the following two blank pages.

Give yourself lots of time to write your obituary so that you can ensure that everything you want to say about yourself is said. If you struggle with writing this yourself, put your information in point form and hire a copywriter to write it out for you or ask your children or a good friend for help.

Spending the time to write our own obituary before we die, is a special opportunity that most people don't take advantage of. Think about it, you know yourself better than anyone else. Writing your own obituary is not only practical, it gives you the chance to express your life story through your own lens, ensuring that the memories and moments that you cherish most are shared exactly as you perceive them.

You may be thinking right now, "Oh, but I can't write." If this is you, don't panic. I can help guide you through the process. In the next few pages you will find some helpful tips for writing your obituary, and a sample of one.

Tips For Writing Your Obituary

Start with the Basics: Begin by listing the fundamental details such as your full name, age, place of birth, and names of close family members.

Reflect on Your Life's Highlights: Consider the significant events, achievements, and turning points in your life. This might include educational achievements, career milestones, hobbies, passions, or impactful travels and experiences. (Refer to your notes in the Reflecting on Your Life chapter, where you have already written many of these things down.)

Share Your Personal Story: Unlike a third-party writing an obituary, you have the unique opportunity to share your life story from your perspective. Mention what you loved, what mattered to you, what you learned, and what you hope to be remembered for.

Include Family and Relationships: Talk about your family and other significant relationships in your life. You may want to express gratitude or love or share special memories.

Discuss Your Values and Beliefs: This can be an opportunity to share the principles and beliefs that guided your life. What did you stand for? What were your passions and causes?

Add Personal Messages: If you wish, include personal messages to your loved ones. This can be a way to say goodbye, offer comfort, or share your hopes for their future. (This will also be covered in The Farewell Message chapter.)

Detail Any Final Wishes: Include any preferences you have for your funeral or memorial service, whether you prefer donations to a specific charity rather than flowers or any other final wishes. (This will be covered in more detail in the My Care and Resting Place Preferences chapter.)

Keep the Tone in Mind: You can choose the tone that suits your personality. It can be sombre, reflective, humorous, straightforward, or a combination of these.

Be Honest and Authentic: Write in a way that truly reflects who you are. This is your final narrative about your life, so make it genuine.

Edit and Review: Make sure to edit and review your obituary. You might even want to share it with someone close to you for feedback. Read through the obituaries in your local newspaper for ideas and find a style that suits you best.

Safekeeping and Accessibility: Ensure that your obituary is stored in a place where it can be easily accessed by your family or executors when needed. You can keep a copy of your obituary right here in between the next two pages of this book, or you can use the pages of this book and have your family refer to this book when handling your affairs.

"Doug died."

Douglas Legler of Fargo, North Dakota,

Sample Self-Authored Obituary

I _____ completed my earthly journey on _____

I was born to _____ and _____ in the year _____

My life has been a tapestry of varied experiences and cherished relationships. From my earliest days in _____ to the milestones that have marked my journey, my life has been filled with noteworthy chapters. I lived for the majority of my life in _____ I remember my days at (school/university/followed by my career(s) and the hobbies that have brought me immense joy, such as

My travels to

and the experiences that I encountered that made me were:

But more than these milestones, what truly defines my life are the relationships and love I've shared.

To my family, (spouse),

(children),

and my beloved (grand children and great grandchildren)

you have been my world. The gratitude and love I feel for you are boundless.

To my friends and those who've walked this journey with me, each of you has left an indelible mark on my heart.

A very special mention to my friends:

Throughout my life, I've held fast to certain values and beliefs primarily:

These principles have guided my decisions and actions, and I hope they continue to inspire even in my absence.

My passions, particularly for

have not only fulfilled me but also, I hope, contributed positively to the world.

As I pen these words, I'd like to leave personal messages for my loved ones.

To

remember that

and to   my hope

for you is:

These words come from the deepest part of my heart, carrying my love and hope for your future.

Here are the details regarding my (celebration/funeral/memorial), and my wish for donations to:

(charity) in lieu of flowers:

In writing my obituary, I've chosen a tone that mirrors my approach to life—perhaps a mix of (reflective/humorous/straightforward).

It's important for me that these words resonate with who I truly was—an individual with flaws and strengths, joys and sorrows, but above all, a heart full of love and a spirit that sought to embrace life fully.

Thank you for being part of my story.

With all my love,

(you)

The Self-Authored Obituary of:

Date:

To whom it may concern, I have authored my obituary. Please fill in the date when it arrives and place this obituary in the following newspapers or online locations after I am gone:

"There are shortcuts to happiness and dancing is one of them!"

Vicki Baum

-4-

The Guest List

When considering one's final arrangements, there are numerous options to choose from, each tailored to individual preferences, beliefs, and circumstances. Traditional funerals, memorial services, elaborate parties, celebrations of life, wakes, private family gatherings, and simple family dinners all offer unique ways to commemorate a loved one's life. Additionally, there are graveside services, cremation services, green burials, direct burials, ash scattering ceremonies, body donation to science, virtual memorial services, living wakes, biographical video tributes, and the incorporation of cultural or religious rituals.

The selection of the appropriate option depends on your wishes and if these aren't made clear then it falls on the shoulders and desires of your loved ones to ensure that your farewell is one that is meaningful and personalized.

Regardless of the type of event that you can choose to honor your life, the personal touches that you add are what transform any type of gathering into a celebration of your life rather than a sombre event. From the attendees to the ambience, music, cuisine, and thematic elements, each detail offers an opportunity to infuse your final occasion with joy and a reflection of your true spirit.

It's in these choices that a gathering about you becomes more than just a typical funeral service that people at times dread attending; it becomes a personalized tribute, a festive gathering that can really tell the true story of who you were to the world.

In this type of celebration, who attends is not determined by wealth, status, or accolades, but by the richness of character, the warmth of heart, and the sincerity of connection.

Crafting the guest list for your event can be a thoughtful and significant part of your celebration planning. It ensures that the people you care about are informed and are sure to attend. I invite you to consider not just who will be present but also the roles these special individuals might play in commemorating your life.

Imagine the faces of friends, family, colleagues, and perhaps even mentors or protégés who have shared in your life's journey. Think about those who have touched your life in meaningful ways and who you wish to be a part of your ultimate celebration.

As you list the names and contact information of the people who you want to make sure attend your celebration, consider the unique connection you share with each person. Reflect on whether there are specific roles or contributions they could make that would add depth and personalization to your event. Perhaps there is someone whose voice would perfectly echo through a cherished song, a dear friend whose words who you know could capture the essence of your journey or a relative whose reading of a favourite poem would resonate with your spirit.

Be as detailed as possible in envisioning how these guests can contribute to making your last hurrah a true reflection of your life, relationships, and the impact you've had on those around you.

It is also critical that you make your wishes known if there is a person or two that you definitely <u>do not want to attend</u> your last hurrah. (*After all, this is your party and you get to invite whomever you wish.*) If you don't want party crashers at your event, make sure to specify in your written obituary that the celebration will be private or you may just attract some unwanted guests. Make sure to mention in your plan for your relatives to discreetly share the information of your celebration if you want to ensure your wishes are respected.

Roles and Responsibilities

Specific roles and responsibilities will be entrusted to those dear friends and cherished family members who have illuminated your life's path.

Below, you'll find the names and designated roles of those who I am hoping will help make this occasion a true reflection of the life I've lived.

Decoration Heads: Decorating the venue in a style that is specified in my plan

Guest Book Attendants: Encouraging guests to write in a memory book to collect stories and messages about me.

Memory Keepers: Curating and displaying photographs or videos to create a visual narrative of my life for guests.

Music Curators: Gathering or performing music that holds significance to me, helping to set the event's tone.

Hospitality Coordinators: Managing event logistics to ensure everything runs smoothly and guests feel comfortable.

Storytellers: Sharing personal anecdotes and memories, offering a heartfelt look into different aspects of my life.

Tribute Leaders: Leading special tributes such as toasts, moments of silence, or meaningful ceremonies.

Food and Beverage Managers: Overseeing catering with dishes or drinks that you list in your plan

Something for you to think about....

Being asked to play a part in your final celebration is a cathartic and meaningful honor for those who love and admire you. Being included in some way, even if it is a small way, allows loved ones to respect you, their relationship with you, your life and legacy, providing them with a sense of personal connection and fulfillment. When people share an experience, like celebrating the life of someone they love, they find support in communal grieving, aiding in their journey of remembrance and healing.

Preplanning the roles people will play in your last hurrah is a gift you can give to others because it is a crucial part of the emotional process of saying goodbye and cherishing the impact you've had on their lives.

"No matter how great a man is, the size of his funeral usually depends on the weather."

Rosemary Clooney

The Guest List

(Names and contact information)

As we age, our relationships and connections with people change and evolve. Creating a living list allows us to reflect on the people who have been important in our lives at different stages and ensure that those who matter to us are written down. Make sure to update this list regularly.

"You know what they say, darling, you can't spell funeral without FUN"

Margo Channing, played by Bette Davis in the 1950 film "All About Eve."

-5-

Crafting the Program

Whether you choose an end-of-life celebration, a funeral, or a private party your theme can still commemorate the joy and love that you brought into the world. These gatherings can all be personalized to reflect your unique life.

Here is a list of fun, creative ways to think about celebrating your life. Read through these and think about how you can infuse vitality into your arrangements.

50 Ways to Leave a *Lasting* Impression

1. **Aerial Salute:** A skywriting message.
2. **Bag Pipes:** Hire a professional bag piper.
3. **Bird/Butterfly Release:** A symbol of peace.
4. **Bubbles:** Environmentally friendly option rather than a balloon release.
5. **Playlist:** Compile a playlist of your favourite songs and have it sent to friends.
6. **Candle Lighting Ceremony:** A candle lighting in a special place at night.
7. **Celebration in Motion:** A guided tour through significant locations in a party bus or train.
8. **Celebratory Parade:** A parade with music, floats, or decorated vehicles.
9. **Community Art Project:** Have a painting party.
10. **Costume Celebration:** Guests dress up in costumes.
11. **Culinary Tour:** A tour through your favorite restaurants.
12. **Cultural Dance Performance:** Featuring a dance form you loved or reflecting your cultural heritage.
13. **Dancing in the Aisle:** Play great music, dance.

14. **Fire Performance:** Fire dancing.
15. **Fishing Party:** Invite your friends to a fishing event.
16. **Flash Mob Tribute:** Organize a surprise performance.
17. **Food and Drink:** Provide a chef prepared meal.
18. **Gun Salute:** 21 Gun Salute.
19. **Home Movie Night:** Compile and view home videos.
20. **Hot Air Balloon Tour:** Hold the entire event up in a hot air balloon with a small group of close friends.
21. **Ice Cream Social:** A fun and sweet way to remember your fondness for ice cream.
22. **Karaoke Celebration:** Set up a karaoke station for guests to sing favourite songs of or related to you.
23. **Kite Flying Event:** A fun family event
24. **Last Wish:** Pre-plan a trip send your surviving spouse around the world. Invite your friends to join.
25. **Legacy Concert:** Give your friends tickets to your favourite concert so they can all go together.
26. **Live Music and Entertainment:** Include live performances or a playlist of your favourite songs.
27. **Memorial Video or Tribute**: Create a pre-recorded video montage with you as the speaker.

28. **Memories and Story Sharing:** Encourage attendees to share memories, stories, or anecdotes about you.
29. **Memory Book or Message Board:** Ask guests to write down memories or messages.
30. **Nature Trail Celebration:** Organize a walk or group hike.
31. **Paddle Out Ceremony:** A Hawaiian tradition, a paddle out in canoes or on surfboards.
32. **Pet-Friendly Gathering:** For the pet lovers
33. **Planting a Tree:** As a living tribute
34. **Poetry Slam or Literary Reading:** Share original poems or read favorite literature excerpts.
35. **Pot Luck Reception:** Ask guests to bring a dish.
36. **Private Concert at Sea:** Charter a yacht or boat and host a private concert at sea.
37. **Recreate an Era:** Example 1950's Costumes.
38. **Rooftop Dinner with Live Opera:** Host a dinner on a rooftop with a live opera performance.
39. **Sand Sculpture Creation:** Creating sand sculptures in your honour at a beach.
40. **Scavenger Hunt:** Organize a scavenger hunt that leads guests through locations significant to your life.

41. **Scuba Divers Dream:** A dive to the coral reef.
42. **Silent Disco:** A personal and interactive dance experience with headphones for guests.
43. **Ski Out:** Ask friends and family to meet on the top of your favourite mountain and do a last run memorial ski, have a beer at the bottom.
44. **Sports Game or Tournament:** Organize a casual game or tournament of your favourite sport.
45. **Star-Naming Ceremony:** Have a star named after you revealing it after your passing.
46. **Social Media Live Tweet:** Guests #hashtag their Instagram photos, or post photos and messages from the service directly onto a memorial Facebook page.
47. **Submarine Tour:** Organize a tour in a submarine and hold the entire ceremony beneath the water.
48. **Time Capsule Creation:** Assemble and bury a time capsule full of memories and photos.
49. **Zen Experience:** Ask guests to bring yoga mats and spend some time in blessings and meditation.
50. **Zero-Gravity Flight Experience:** Organize a zero-gravity flight to symbolize freedom and the spirit of exploration.

Simple is Also Good

In the midst of elaborate memorials, there's a unique beauty in simplicity as well.

A close friend, a lover of light beer and the serenity of riverside camping with her family, valued simple pleasures in life. For her farewell gathering, she dreamed about inviting all who knew her to the river's edge, where under the open sky, on a warm summer evening, everyone would crack open cold beers, toasting not only her memory but also the embodiment of her values and the person she had been. Sometimes, the most meaningful memorials are those that echo the unadorned purity of one's spirit and the authenticity of their passions. Cheers to a life well-lived and the extraordinary beauty found in simplicity.

Note to the Reader

Whatever you choose, be sure to verify and obtain the necessary permits for any plan you want to put in place and always consider the environment, avoiding options that may harm it.

Now It's Your Turn

After exploring these diverse and creative ways to celebrate a life, it's time to reflect on what resonates most with you. Each of us has different elements that we hold dear, and your celebration should be a reflection of you and what makes your heart sing.

A week before he died in 2022, Oprah Winfrey threw a going away party in a backyard for her dying father, Vernon Winfrey. What a privilege it must have been for her to be able to gift him this special celebration of his life. This living wake picnic also gave Oprah's father the opportunity to say good-bye to all of his friends, share old memories and get together one last time. A living wake is also one way of celebrating your life and something to think about.

What elements do you feel are the most important to be included in your last hurrah celebration? Is it the music? How about the speeches or the food? Do you want dancing or singing? A simple ceremony by a river, or a huge party? There is so much to think about !!

Why don't we begin by writing (in point form) a list of a few things that you feel are most *important for* you to have incorporated into your last hurrah. Begin with your #1 most most important element and go down from there.

The most important element of my last hurrah is: (food, music, entertainment, theme, guest list, speeches, etc.)

Where would you like the event to be held? A traditional funeral home? A rented hall? A private home? A park? The beach? In a forest? Does a living wake interest you?

Here is a list of my favorite songs that I would like to be played at my last hurrah.

Copyright Considerations*: If your celebration is a private event, playing recorded music generally won't require special permissions. However, if the event is public or being broadcasted, such as in a live stream, be mindful of copyright issues. Using royalty-free music or obtaining the necessary permissions is advisable in these cases.*

I would like to have the following live entertainment (include specifics, if possible, such as the names and phone numbers of musicians, singers, etc.):

_____

_____

_____

_____

I would like to include the following food/drinks:

I would like to have the following theme, decorations, colors, flowers and ambience:

Throughout life, certain rituals and traditions hold special places in our hearts, weaving together the essence of who we are and what we believe in. These rituals and traditions can be incorporated into our final celebration whether they are born from religious or personal convictions. These are mine:

Writing Your Eulogy

A eulogy, is an integral part of a memorial service, and it can be delivered by various individuals including close family members, friends, religious or spiritual leaders, or professional officiants. A Eulogy is a weaving of personal stories and heartfelt tributes to honor you. You can have someone write it for you, after you pass or you can write your own before you go. You can also record your eulogy and have it played for everyone to hear.

The approach of writing your own, not only allows you to reflect on your life and the legacy you wish to leave but also offers a final, meaningful message to your loved ones, ensuring your thoughts and feelings are shared exactly as you intend.

Whether delivered by someone close to you or crafted by your own hand, a eulogy is a powerful tool for remembrance and closure, connecting the audience through shared memories and emotions.

Note to the Reader

If you find resonance with the following self authored eulogy and feel it reflects your thoughts and feelings, please feel free to use it as your own. You can personalize it by adding specific anecdotes, memories, or messages that are unique to your life and experiences.

If you prefer to have this done for you, you may consider hiring a professional eulogy writer.

Check out <u>eulogyassistant.com</u>

Once written, your eulogy can then serve as a heartfelt farewell message to your loved ones, capturing your essence and leaving a lasting impression of your journey and the love you shared.

Sample Self Authored Eulogy

As I write this, I'm filled with a sense of gratitude. Gratitude for the life I've lived, for the people who've filled it with love, and for the moments both big and small that have made up the tapestry of my existence.

I've always believed life is a beautiful journey with its share of ups and downs. And like any good story, it's not just the destination that matters, but the journey itself – the experiences, the laughter, the tears, and most importantly, the people who shared it with us.

To my wonderful family, thank you for your unending love and support. You have been my rock, my guiding light, and my greatest blessing. The memories we've created together are the treasures I carried in my heart.

To my dear friends, thank you for the joy, the adventures, and even the ridiculous moments. Each of you added colour and vibrancy to my life. Our friendships were the threads that helped hold the fabric of my life together.

I hope I've left you with happy memories and stories to tell. I hope I've made you laugh more than I've made you cry. And above all, I hope I've shown you the importance of love, kindness, and the value of a life well-lived.

Please don't remember me with sadness. Instead, celebrate the time we had, the love we shared, and the impact we had on each other's lives. Sing the songs I loved, share the stories that make you smile, and live your lives with the same joy and passion that I tried to live mine.

I leave you with no regrets, just a wish that I had more time to enjoy the beautiful world we live in. But I've had a fulfilling life, and for that, I am eternally grateful.

So, as I say goodbye, remember that in every sunrise, in every laughter, in every beautiful thing you see, a part of me is there, smiling with you.

My Self Authored Eulogy

My Name is: _____

To be read by: _____

With all my love,

"Do not go gentle into that good night, Old age should burn and rave at close of day; Rage, rage against the dying light."

Dylan Thomas

The Last Hurrah Party Plan

Take a moment to revisit all the insightful answers you've provided to the questions in the workbook thus far. Afterward, read the sample 'Last Hurrah Plan' in the next few pages. Utilize the combined insights from your own answers and the sample plan to refine and finalize the details of Your Last Hurrah Plan. Let the fun begin…

Sample Last Hurrah Plan

Theme: A Journey Through Your Life

A theme that encapsulates the essence of your life journey, reflecting your personality, passions, and experiences.

Location: [A Meaningful Place]Choose a location that holds special significance to you, such as a favourite park, beach, garden, or even a family home.

Date and Time: Select a date that is meaningful or convenient for family and friends, possibly around a birthday, an anniversary, or a significant family date.

Welcome and Introduction: A close friend or family member opens the celebration with a warm welcome.

Music and Performances: Live music featuring your favourite songs or genres. Performances by local musicians or recordings of your favourite artists.

Memory Sharing: Invited guests share stories, anecdotes, and memories of you. A microphone is passed around for anyone who wishes to speak.

Photo and Memorabilia Display: A photo montage or slideshow showcasing moments of your life. Tables displaying memorabilia, awards, artwork, or personal items.

Readings of favourite poems, quotes, or literature. Family members or friends may read letters or messages from you.

A group activity that reflects hobbies or interests, such as planting a tree, releasing lanterns, or a group art project.

Meal and Toasts: A meal or a buffet featuring your favourite dishes and drinks. Toasts in honour of celebrating your life and legacy.

Farewell Ritual: A symbolic gesture to say goodbye, such as a balloon release, candle lighting, or a moment of silence

Keepsakes for Guests: Custom keepsakes or mementos for guests to take home, such as a crystal with your name on it to hang in their window, a small booklet of your favourite recipes, a book of poems, a custom bookmark, or a package of seeds of your favourite flower.

Closing Remarks: Final words by close family members or friends, thanking guests for their love and support.

Details For My Last Hurrah Plan

Location:

Date and Time: (evening or daytime)

Theme: (decorations, dress-code, flowers, atmosphere)

Welcome and Introduction: (names and contact info)

Music and Performance: (names and contact info)

Memory Sharing: (names or open mic)

Photo and Memorabilia display: (video presentation, photos, poems, placed on a table or in a handout)

Food and drinks: (before, during or at an after party)

Toasts and the Final Farewell Ritual: (balloons, doves, a dance party, candle lighting, or a hug fest)

Keepsakes for Guests: (closing remarks or your farewell speech read out or pre-recorded for everyone to listen to)

The most important elements of my celebration are:

"See you later, alligator"

Bill Haley through his song "See You Later, Alligator," released in 1955.

-6-
Writing Your Farewell Message

Writing your own farewell message or letter is a deeply personal and poignant opportunity to express your feelings, thoughts, and reflections.

A farewell message is different from a eulogy. A eulogy, even if authored by you, gives a narrative of your life from an external viewpoint, focusing on your achievements as a tribute to all that you have done and enjoyed throughout your life.

Your farewell message allows you to directly communicate your final thoughts and feelings, providing a deeply personal touch to your ceremony.

A farewell message is a chance for you to say your final goodbyes or to communicate what might not have been said during your lifetime and to leave parting words that can provide closure, comfort, and lasting memories for those you care about.

Your farewell message can be delivered as a pre-recorded message or read out by someone close to you at the beginning of your celebration, your dinner or before the festivities begin. It is your one last chance to tell everyone how much you love them and want them to enjoy themselves at your spectacular last hurrah.

Tips for Writing your Farewell Message

Begin with Reflection: Start by reflecting on your life, the relationships you've had, and the experiences that have shaped you. Think about the people who have been significant in your life and what you'd like to say to them.

Express Gratitude: One of the most powerful elements in a farewell speech or letter is expressing gratitude. Thank those who have been part of your journey for their love, support, and the moments you've shared.

Share Memories and Stories: Include personal anecdotes or stories that are meaningful to you and those you are addressing. These stories can bring comfort and smiles and help keep your memory alive.

Be Honest, but Gentle: While honesty is important, it's also crucial to approach sensitive topics with gentleness and consideration. The goal is to leave a positive impact, not to settle scores.

Offer Forgiveness and Seek it if Needed: If there are relationships that involve hurt or misunderstanding, consider offering forgiveness. Similarly, if you feel you may have wronged others, this could be an opportunity to apologize and seek reconciliation.

Share Your Hopes for Loved Ones: Include your hopes and wishes for those you're leaving behind. This can be particularly comforting for family and friends, as it shows your love and care for their future well-being.

Include Personal Sign-offs: Personalize messages for specific individuals if it feels appropriate. These tailored goodbyes can be very meaningful to the recipients.

Reflect Your Personality: Let your speech or letter reflect your personality. Whether it's through humor, wisdom, or storytelling, it should sound like you.

Ask for what you need: Consider asking your loved ones to continue on with the causes you care about by writing letters to Congress in support of work you are passionate about, ask people to recycle and work towards protecting the planet.

Offer Comfort: Remember, this letter or speech is not just for you but also for those you leave behind. Aim to provide comfort, closure, and peace.

Final Thoughts: End with final thoughts that encapsulate your view of life, your gratitude, or your love. This could be a quote, a personal philosophy, or a simple expression of love and goodbye.

"How lucky am I to have something that makes saying goodbye so hard."

Winnie the Pooh

My Farewell Message

This is a special spot for you to leave private letters and notes for those closest to you

Personal Notes and Private Letters

118

"I can't afford to die; I'd lose too much money."

George Burns

-7-

The Practicalities of Parting

An essential yet often overlooked aspect of life's final arrangements is the business end. I know, it's boring and not as fun as planning your party but it will help your family immensely. The practical part helps ensure a smooth transition and lessening the burden on your loved ones during a time of grief.

Where There's A Will There's A Way

I am assuming that you have your Last Will and Testament written and held in a safe place. If you don't have a Will, PLEASE get one drawn up today.

Dying without a Will, known legally as dying 'intestate,' can lead to complex and often unintended consequences for your loved ones. Without a Will, you lose control over who inherits your assets and how things are distributed. The laws of the state or country will determine this, and the process can be lengthy, stressful, and costly for your family. It can also lead to potential conflicts among relatives and might not reflect your personal wishes or the needs of your beneficiaries.

Creating a Will is a crucial step in ensuring that your assets are distributed according to your desires and that your loved ones are provided for in the way you intend. It's a significant part of estate planning that offers peace of mind, clarity, and a smooth transition for those you care about most.

In this day and age, creating a Will is simpler than ever. You can either create a Will in person with a lawyer or you can create one online in the comfort of your easy chair. Right now if you like.

Here are a few on-line resources to check out :

In Canada: Willful, LegalWills.ca, LawDepot.

In the USA: LegalZoom, Rocket Lawyer.

The next most important thing, after you have written and signed your will of course, is to store it in a secure location and remember where you put it.

This next chapter is the perfect place for you to record and organize all of the critical information that the people you leave behind will need such as where your Will is located and who to contact. This information is invaluable and will help make a fairly difficult process much easier for everyone involved. Your foresight in these matters will be the final act of love and consideration, valued and remembered by your family.

Dearest loved ones,

Here, let me make things easier for you…..

Important Documents

My Will is located:

Address:

Estate Lawyer's Name:

Contact:

My Executor is:

Contact Number:

Notes:

There is a loose protocol for notifying individuals when someone has passed away. This typically starts with immediate family members learning of the news first, followed by close friends and relatives. While this protocol offers a general framework, it's essential for families to take into account their unique circumstances, cultural practices, and the preferences of the deceased when informing loved ones of the loss.

Note to the Reader *Please keep the communication compassionate, timely, and respectful during this sensitive time.*

Please contact immediately:

Names					Phone Numbers

My Important Contacts List:

Include a list of other important contacts such as your business attorneys, financial advisors, insurance agents, bank managers, and any other professionals who have been involved in your estate planning and management.

Name   Phone Number

Bank Accounts: Include a list of the banks and addresses of the branches where you have accounts, plus the account numbers, type of account, etc.

Investments and Retirement Funds / Pension Fund/ Insurance Policies, Social Security Income Information:

Social insurance number and tax accountant's information: Include a copy of your last income tax return for easy reference.

Safety deposit box/storage locker locations: Tape your well-labelled keys here or write down where you keep them.

Real Estate and Other Significant Assets:

Vehicle Information: Include information about where the titles are stored/insurance documents are and any loan or lease information. (*Or better yet, place a photocopy of these documents right here, between the pages of this book.*)

Debts and Liabilities:

Household account numbers: Include an envelope with copies of each current bill for easy access, such as telephone, hydro, gas, house taxes, car insurance, etc.

Digital Footprint:

List online identities and passwords, for posthumous account management or deletion. Here are some to consider:

Blogs and personal websites.

Cloud storage accounts.

Digital photo and video libraries.

Email accounts.

Gaming profiles

Medical records.

Online banking

PayPal

Photos stored in iCloud.

Important Passwords

Mobile Phone Password:

Computer Passwords:

Social Media Profiles :

Others:

Keys and Access Information: If there are codes, or other access information needed to access your home.

Include a copy of the following documents between these pages or their whereabouts here:

1. Your Birth Certificate.

2. Your Marriage and Divorce Certificates.

3. Passport/Citizenship or Resident Card.

4. Drivers License.

Location Notes:

Taking the initiative to organize and document the business aspects of your life is a thoughtful and valuable gift to your loved ones. Beyond being an act of goodwill, it serves as a proactive measure to bring peace of mind to both you and your family. By doing so, you streamline the process of handling the administrative and paperwork aspects that come with end-of-life matters. This thoughtful preparation can ease the burden on your family during an already challenging time, making the transition smoother and more straightforward.

Remember, the goal is not only to provide direction but also to convey your care and consideration in making their journey through this difficult time a little easier.

Note to the Reader

By the time you have completed this chapter you will definitely need to store this book in a secure place with all your other important documents. Place this in your safety deposit box or wherever you keep your important papers, such as your Last Will and Testament.

"I wish I'd done more housework while I was alive"

said no tombstone ever.

-8-

Care and Resting Place Preferences

In my own experience, and from what others have told me, one crucial thing that families often wish their loved ones had done, besides having a will, is to leave clear instructions about their end-of-life preferences. This includes details about their funeral arrangements and how they want to be remembered. It's a topic that's frequently discussed in estate planning and is often highlighted in articles and studies focusing on end-of-life planning. Knowing whether a loved one preferred a traditional funeral or something more personal, or even their choice of music and readings, can significantly lessen the burden on families during a difficult time. It brings a sense of relief and certainty, ensuring that they're honoring their loved one's wishes in the way they intended.

The next few pages are dedicated to outlining your preferences for end-of-life care and final wishes regarding the handling of your physical remains, whether through burial or cremation. Deciding on these matters in advance and communicating them <u>clearly</u> to your family is a crucial step in easing the burden on loved ones during a time of deep emotion and grief. It's not just about making choices; it's about ensuring that one's values, beliefs, and preferences are respected and followed at the end of your life.

Some helpful terms

The following terms will help you and your loved ones make informed decisions together about your end-of-life care and ensure that your wishes are respected. It's important to also discuss these terms with your healthcare providers and possibly an attorney to ensure that <u>all legal documents are properly executed and reflect your desires.</u>

An Advance Healthcare Directive: All documents that express your healthcare preferences in advance. It includes not only a document called a Living Will but also other directives, such as the appointment of a healthcare proxy or power of attorney for healthcare. The person you authorize will be able to make medical decisions on your behalf in the event that you are unable to do so yourself.

A Living Will: A document that is part of detailing your preferences for medical treatment, including end-of-life care, in situations where you are unable to communicate. It often outlines conditions under which you would or would not want life-sustaining treatments.

(DNR) order: This means "Do Not Resuscitate." It is a directive to medical personnel not to perform CPR or advanced life support if your heart stops or if you stop breathing, which can be part of a Living Will or advance directive, reflecting your wishes for specific emergency medical situations.

Death Doula: A person that assists families living with imminent death. Death doulas offer non-medical, compassionate support to you and your family as you go through the dying process.

Healthcare Power of Attorney (POA): A legal document that designates a person to make healthcare decisions on your behalf if you are unable to do so.

Care Preferences: An outline of your preferences for end-of-life care. This might include your thoughts on hospice care, pain management, and anything above, including the type of medical interventions you would or would not like to receive. There are specific medical forms that serve to communicate your preferences for life-sustaining treatments across various healthcare settings, ensuring that your end-of-life care aligns with their wishes. Discuss this with your physician.

Palliative Care: This type of care focuses on relieving the symptoms and stress of serious illness, regardless of the diagnosis. The goal is to improve quality of life for you and your family.

Hospice Care: Hospice is a form of palliative care specifically designed for end-of-life situations when a patient is generally considered to have six months or less to live and has chosen to forego curative treatments.

Organ and Tissue Donation: You should discuss organ and tissue donation with your family, healthcare provider, and legal advisor to ensure your wishes are known and respected.

Ethical Will: This is not a legal document but a personal letter that expresses your thoughts, values, life lessons, and hopes for the future, often shared with family and friends. There is a space for you to write your own Ethical Will in the final chapter of this book.

Note to Reader

Some of the arrangements mentioned on the prior pages require legal documents that need to be prepared before they are needed and discussed with family members, healthcare proxies, and physicians to ensure everyone understands your wishes. It's important to consult with a healthcare provider and a legal expert in your specific jurisdiction to understand the exact requirements and process for initiating specific orders such as a DNR order. The laws and regulations governing DNR orders can vary significantly between different regions and countries.

Valuable Resources:

Five Wishes: The Five Wishes document is an advance directive that helps adults of all ages specify their preferences for medical, personal, emotional, and spiritual care if they become seriously ill and are unable to communicate. It serves as a comprehensive guide for end-of-life planning. For details or to obtain the document, visit Aging with Dignity's official website:

fivewishes.org or agingwithdignity.org

Advance Care Planning: (Canada) For resources and guidance on the Advance Care Planning in Canada visit advancecareplanning.ca and dyingwithdignity.ca

National Institute on Aging: (USA) For free worksheets for end-of-life decision making visit: nia.nih.gov

My Thoughts On End-Of-Life Care:

Living Will/Directive: If you have a Living Will, or an advance healthcare directive, a DNR provide details about where these documents are located.

Healthcare Proxy or Power of Attorney: Identify who you have designated as your healthcare proxy or who holds your medical power of attorney. This person will make healthcare decisions for you if you are unable to do so yourself. Provide details about where this document is located.

Burial (Natural or Traditional) or Cremation

Burial or cremation are two common but different ways of handling our bodies. Burial involves interring the body in the ground or a mausoleum, often in a casket, and is chosen for various personal, cultural, or religious reasons.

Cremation, on the other hand, incinerates a body to ashes, offering a more cost-effective option with greater flexibility for memorial services and the handling of remains.

The choice between the two usually depends on individual preferences, beliefs, and financial factors.

The other option is a natural burial which is an eco-friendly approach to laying a person to rest. In a natural burial chemical preservation is avoided which minimizes the use of non-biodegradable materials. In essence, you are not embalmed and typically buried in a simple, biodegradable casket or shroud, or sometimes directly in the earth. It involves the manual digging of the grave and the use of natural methods for preparing the body. The final resting place is often marked with unobtrusive markers like natural stones or a planted tree, rather than traditional headstones, ensuring a minimal environmental impact.

Choosing how you want your body to be handled after you pass spares the people that are left the emotional weight of making such a choice during a time of grief.

I'm sure by this time in your life you have given this some thought and preplanning ensures your wishes are followed. It also prevents potential conflicts among family members, making the process smoother during a very difficult period.

This one act of pre-arrangement is a considerate way to reduce stress for your loved ones another intangible gift you will be can leave for your loved ones.

My Burial Plan

If you have pre-arranged and pre-paid for your burial, funeral or cremation service please provide the details here:

_____

_____

If not, these are my wishes.

I would like to be buried/ or cremated/ natural burial

_____

_____

_____

Signature: _____

Burial: If you prefer burial, provide details such as the type of burial (natural or traditional) . If having a traditional burial in a cemetery, specify the preferred cemetery, the type of casket, and whether you have already purchased a plot (if so, include where it is located). If it is a natural burial you prefer, write that down. In both instances write where you would like to be buried.

Cremation: Cremation has emerged as a popular choice, valued for its simplicity and environmental friendliness. The resulting ashes, often referred to as cremated remains, are carefully placed into an urn or a selected container. Cremation resonates with those who appreciate its eco-friendly attributes and versatility as an end-of-life option.

Thinking Outside of the Box

Beyond its practicality, there's also a world of creative possibilities for those seeking unique and even whimsical ways to memorialize your ashes. The range of creative options adds a layer of meaningful and even fun possibilities to the process. Have you ever thought of becoming a tree or even a diamond? What about being mixed with paint and becoming a painting of yourself by one of your favorite artists?

Creative Ways to Memorialize Your Ashes

- **Hourglass:** Use ashes to fill an hourglass as a symbol of ongoing life.

- **Birdhouse Installation:** Place ashes in a birdhouse to create a living memorial with nature.

- **Bio Tree Urn:** Designed to turn you into a tree after you are gone.

- **Bonsai Tree:** Grow a bonsai tree with ashes in the soil, symbolizing life's continuity.

- **Candle:** Craft a candle with ashes, offering a comforting source of light.

- **Coral Reef Contribution:** Add ashes to an artificial reef to support marine life.

- **Commemorative Bookmark:** Embed ashes into a handmade bookmark.

- **Commemorative Pottery:** Incorporate ashes into clay for pottery or ceramics.

- **Cremation Garden:** Bury ashes in a dedicated garden.

- **Customized Memorial Bench:** Construct a bench with a compartment for ashes.

- **Diamond:** Transform ashes into a diamond.

- **Distributed Memorial:** Share ashes among various places or family members.

- **Dove Release:** Place ashes in a small bio-degradable container and set them free.

- **Forest Planting:** Mixing ashes with soil to grow a living tree memorial.

- **Fountain Pen:** Create a fountain pen with a capsule containing ashes in the barrel.

- **Garden Sculpture:** Place ashes in a garden sculpture to merge art with nature.

- **Garden Steppingstones:** Create personalized stones with ashes.

- **Glass Keepsake Box:** Store ashes in a glass keepsake box with sentimental designs.

- **Glass Sculpture:** Ashes infused in to any shape

- **Green Burial:** An eco-friendly way to return to the earth by dispersing ashes in a beloved location rivers, park, ocean, forest, mountains. (check by-laws).

- **Handwritten Script Memorial:** Use ink mixed with ashes for meaningful messages.

- **Home Memorial:** Keep ashes in a decorative urn at home, such as a teapot.

- **Incorporation into Art:** Turn ashes into various forms of artwork.

- **Keepsake:** Locket or ring .

- **Northern Lights Cremation Urn:** (Aurora Borealis.)

- **Ocean Reef:** Contribute ashes to create an artificial reef, supporting ocean ecosystems.

- **Painting:** Mix ashes with paint and have an artist create a custom piece of artwork.

- **Puzzle:** Craft a jigsaw puzzle featuring an image created with ashes.

- **Paperweight:** Rainbow bridge memorial glass

- **Sand Art:** Use ashes to create intricate sand art designs.

- **Seeds:** Have ashes mixed with wildflower seeds.

- **Sculpture:** Place ashes in a garden sculpture to merge art with nature.

- **Skydiver Scatter :** Ashes to be spread in the free fall. *check by-laws

- **Space Travel:** Get sent into orbit.

- **Stained Glass Window:** Embedding ashes into stained glass for a luminous memory.

- **Snow Globe:** Using ashes.

- **Sun catcher:** Embed ashes into a crystal and have it made into a sun-catcher.

- **Tattoo:** Mix ashes with tattoo ink for a lasting tribute.

- **Teddy Bear Urn:** Stuffed inside a stuffy.

- **Time Capsule:** Sealing ashes in a time capsule for future discovery.

- **Trip around the world:** Plan the itinerary and have your loved ones take your ashes in their suitcase. *check laws

- **Vinyl Record:** Having ashes pressed into a vinyl record to play memories in music.

- **Water Burial:** Submerge a biodegradable urn containing ashes in a body of water.

- **Wind Chime:** Fashion a wind chime with ashes-infused materials for soothing melodies.

Vessels for Ashes

Urns come in all shapes and sizes. I recently saw an urn in the shape of a Viking Long Boat, supposedly created for those who want a send off to remember.

Why not leave one less decision to your grieving family and choose the final vessel yourself. Pick a unique urn or container for ashes that reflects your personality and interests. (Wood, ceramic, glass, metal, stone). Choose the shape and size of your urn. There are also bio-degradable urns available for ocean burials and green burials.

There are hundreds of different scattering tubes available for sale on Amazon if you choose to have your ashes scattered. A scattering tube is not for storing ashes in, its for transportation of the ashes to the scattering spot. The tube can be biodegradable, bamboo, painted with a theme, decorated, wooden, compact and travel-friendly.

Specifics of Cremation: If you prefer cremation, provide details such as where you want you would like to be cremated, and what you would like to have done with your ashes.

Note to Reader

Before proceeding with any scattering ceremony, it's crucial to thoroughly research and confirm the applicable laws and obtain any necessary permits to ensure a respectful and legal memorialization process.

It's crucial to check the specific airline and country regulations before you travel to ensure that you comply with all requirements. Additionally, consider contacting the airline directly to clarify their policies and procedures for transporting ashes on their flights.

"It's awfully dark in here. "

Jane Doe

Ash Transportation: I would like my ashes to be placed in a scattering tube like the following: (Describe the type or provide a picture if necessary)

Ash Preservation (if not scattered): If I do not wish for my ashes to be scattered, please follow these instructions: (Specify your preservation preferences here.)

Urns (if applicable): I would prefer my ashes to be stored in an urn with the following characteristics: (Describe the urn's shape, material, and any other specific details.)

Ash Disposition: Regarding my ashes, I would like the following to be done: (Explain your wishes for what should be done with your ashes.)

_____

_____

_____

_____

Date:_____

Signature:_____

Words That Last - Your Epitaph

An epitaph is a meaningful inscription of words, often etched into tombstones or memorial markers. These markers are crafted from a diverse array of materials, including enduring options like granite, elegant choices like marble, durable bronze plaques, as well as practical materials like concrete and natural stones such as slate and limestone. Once written, your epitaph can be transcribed, fastened or carved onto an urn, benches, placed on a plaque beneath trees, or on a vessel of your choice. The selection of the material you place your epitaph on depends on your preference, budget, and often cemetery regulations.

Once you choose the material, the epitaph is carefully created, either through meticulous carving, precise engraving, or other suitable methods. In this way, your epitaph becomes a lasting tribute, preserving your memory and your legacy for generations to come.

Choose your words carefully as your epitaph will be inscribed on your tombstone or plaque for years to come. This is another unique opportunity for you to leave a lasting expression of your personality, beliefs, or humor that speaks beyond life.

Writing your own epitaph is a choice, an intimate way to contribute to your own legacy and to impart a final message that reflects who you are or what you stood for.

Don't worry if you can't decide exactly what to say right now, jot down a few that you like. One of the benefits of a living workbook like this is that it allows you to make updates along the way.

Take your time writing your epitaph, knowing that it may change as you do, but having something written down now is a great way to start. Allow your last words to be a true reflection of who you are at this moment in time and also of the life you've lived up until now, encapsulating your essence in a few, carefully chosen words.

The upcoming pages are brimming with both common and even a handful of outrageously creative epitaphs.

Writing an epitaph can be a profoundly cathartic journey, and as you go back through your journal entries you may discover a few gems that perfectly capture the essence of who you are and what your ultimate parting words should be.

50 Common Sign Offs

1. A Life Full of Years, Not Regrets.
2. A Life Well Lived.
3. A Loving Father/Mother/Husband/Wife.
4. A True Gentleman/Lady.
5. Always in Our Thoughts.
6. Always Loved and Remembered.
7. An Inspiration to All.
8. Beloved by All Who Knew Him/Her.

9. Cherished Memories Never Fade.

10. Deeply Loved, Forever Missed.

11. Endlessly Loved and Missed.

12. Eternally Loved and Remembered.

13. Forever in Our Hearts.

14. Forever Missed, Never Forgotten.

15. Gone But Never Forgotten.

16. Gone from Our Lives, but Never Our Hearts.

17. In Eternal Sleep.

18. In Loving Memory.

19. Life's Work Well Done.

20. Love, Laughter, Friendship.

21. Loved and Remembered Every Day.

22. Loving Memories Last Forever.

23. Memories Cherished.

24. Missed Beyond Measure.

25. Never Far from Our Thoughts.

26. Never Forgotten, Forever Loved.
27. Our Beloved (Name).
28. Peace at Last.
29. Resting in Peace and Love.
30. Sadly Missed by All.
31. So Dearly Loved, So Sadly Missed.
32. The Heart of Our Family.
33. The Light of Our Lives.
34. Till Memory Fades and Life Departs.
35. Time Passes, Love Remains.
36. Together in the Same Old Way.
37. Too Dearly Loved to Be Forgotten.
38. Treasured Memories.
39. Until We Meet Again.
40. We Will Always Love You.
41. With a Smile in Our Hearts.
42. Your Love Lights Our Way.

43. Your Memory Lives On.

44. A Gentle Soul, Forever in Our Hearts.

45. A Life Measured in Love, Not Years.

46. Always Our Hero.

47. Beyond the Sunset.

48. Forever Young at Heart.

49. Laughter, Joy, Friendship.

50. Love is Eternal.

Humorous Epitaphs

1. "Turn me over, I'm done on this side." Lawrence of Rome, Deacon

2. "And now for a final word from our sponsor" Charles Gussman, Radio and TV Announcer.

3. "I told you I was ill." Spike Milligan

4. "Here lies John Yeast. Pardon me for not rising."

5. "I'd rather be in Philadelphia." WC Fields

6. In a twist of poetic irony, "Here lies Ezra Pound, lost at sea and never found" (fictional)

7. Enjoy the view.

8. She was an acquired taste.

9. Now I know.

10. Finally got my own park bench.

11. Best seat in the house, and it's all mine!

12. Sit down, relax, I've been expecting you!

13. Taking a long pause in my favourite place.

14. Benchwarmer extraordinaire, at your service.

15. Rest here and chat with me awhile.

16. Watching the world go by, care to join?

17. Here for the stories and the sunshine.

18. Always loved a good view, now I share mine.

19. This bench is my final masterpiece.

20. Time to go.

21. It never hurts to keep looking for sunshine.

I want to have my Epitaph written on this material:

(Granite, stone, brass plaque, urn)

I want my Epitaph to be placed at this location:

My Epitaph:

Beyond Goodbye

Gifts from beyond the grave hold a special, poignant significance, allowing one's legacy and love to endure even after passing. These thoughtful preparations can take many forms, each infused with deep personal meaning. Consider a series of handwritten letters, each to be opened on specific future dates or milestones, offering love, advice, or simply cherished memories. Another touching gesture could be setting up a fund or savings account for a loved one's education or dream project, a testament to your belief in their future. For those who appreciate a more tangible connection, a piece of jewelry or a treasured personal item can become a cherished heirloom, carrying with it stories and memories. Some choose to record video messages or voice recordings, creating a lasting presence in their loved ones' lives.

Pre-planning such gifts reflect a deep care and foresight, a way to continue participating in the lives of those you hold dear, even in absence.

1. Collection of personal stories or life lessons compiled into a book for loved ones,(like this book.)

2. Commissioned piece of art that embodies your spirit or commemorates your life.

3. Custom playlist of songs that hold special meaning, to be shared with loved ones.

4. Donation to a cherished charity in your name.

5. "Memory quilt" made from your clothes or personal fabrics for your family.

6. Prepaid flower delivery for special occasions for a year after you are gone.

7. Pre-paid funeral or cremation.

8. Leave a recipe book of your favourite dishes for family and friends.

9. Scholarship fund set up in your memory for students in need.

10. Trust fund for your children's or grandchildren's education.

11. Video or voice recording or pre-written anniversary and birthday cards

Dressed to Impress: My Going Away Outfit

Did you know that choosing what a loved one should wear for their final goodbye is undoubtedly one of the top most emotionally taxing decisions a family can face? Most families wish their departed loved ones had taken care of this in advance.

Grief already weighs heavily during such times, and having to make seemingly small yet significant choices like this can intensify the emotional burden.

When someone passes away, the people left behind earnestly are struggling as they strive to honor your wishes. Choosing your outfit can feel overwhelming amidst the grieving process. Family dynamics come into play, with each member having their own opinions, which can further complicate the decision-making process.

By making these decisions in advance, you're not just being practical; you're providing a tremendous source of relief for your family. It's a lot easier for our loved ones to follow explicit instructions such as, 'dress me in my beloved pink dress' than struggle through tears and uncertainty while trying to guess what you might have liked.

Let's face it, its always hard to think of what to wear to any event. Your own funeral is no exception. Deciding what to wear to the biggest party of your life is something that you can do right now. Take some time to select the perfect outfit that shows you off in your best light.

Your outfit can be as casual as flip-flops and a Hawaiian shirt, or as formal as a wedding dress. Its one hundred percent up to you.

Don't forget the accessories! Do you have a treasured piece of jewelry, a watch perhaps? Alongside your outfit, you can include any items of emotional significance: heartfelt letters from loved ones, a few favourite photographs from memorable events like your wedding, or small meaningful things such as your favourite poetry book.

Your choices should reflect your style. By taking a few moments to jot down these wishes before hand ensures that your final farewell is one that is deeply personal and reflective of the life you've lived, providing comfort and a sense of closeness to those you leave behind.

Preparing in advance isn't just about personalizing your farewell; it's also a gesture of comfort and closure for your loved ones.

Picking out your last outfit ahead of time may seem like a small step, but it is huge and significantly reduces stress during an already challenging period.

"Life is a party. Dress like it."

Audrey Hepburn

My Final Outfit

Dress me in this:

_____

_____

_____

_____

_____

Things I want to take with me : (photos, jewelry, phone etc)

_____

_____

Date:_____   Signature:_____

The last chapter of your life

has not been written yet.

You hold the pen.

-9-

The Final Chapter

As we journey through the pages of life, each chapter we write is a unique blend of joys, challenges, triumphs, and transformations. This chapter is your canvas, a sacred space where you can paint a picture of who you truly are beyond the roles and responsibilities that have defined you. It's a chance to pause and ask yourself: When the final curtain falls, how do I want to be remembered? What message do I wish to leave behind for the world?

Life is a dynamic, ever-evolving journey. Just as seasons change, so do we. This chapter, like the pages of this book, is not static; this is a living document that grows and matures as you do. Here, you have the freedom to express your deepest values, the lessons you've cherished, the love you've given and received, and the unique footprint you wish to leave on the sands of time.

In these final pages, take a moment to reflect. When the final curtain falls on the stage of your life, how would you like people to remember you? What message should endure for the world to hold onto?

An Ethical Will is a document that you can write to record the message you want to leave to the world. Your Last Will and Testament is a legal document, an Ethical Will is not a legal document, but a document that expresses your values, beliefs, blessings, and advice for future generations, rather than material possessions.

Before you begin to write your Ethical Will, take a few moments to go back through the answers that you've been writing in this workbook. Think about all the moments that have shaped you, the dreams you've pursued, and the legacy you aim to create.

An Ethical Will is an opportunity for you to tell your story in your own words and share your wisdom, insights, and hopes. It's a chance to tell the world about the causes you hold dear, the passions that ignite your spirit, and the memories you want to be remembered by—what your thoughts are on life.

How do you want to be remembered? Is it for your kindness, your courage, your creativity, or your unwavering commitment to the things you believe in? What are the stories, anecdotes, and philosophies that encapsulate your essence?

Your Ethical Will is the perfect platform for you to articulate all of this.

As you pen down your thoughts, remember that this is not just an exercise in reminiscing but a powerful tool in shaping your legacy. It's a testament to your journey, a beacon for those you'll someday leave behind, and a guiding light for future generations. Take your time and think them through.

12 Questions To Help You Get Started.

1. What principles and values have guided my life's decisions, and how can I pass these on as a moral compass for my descendants?

2. Which personal experiences have offered crucial insights that I consider essential to share with the next generation

3. Can I identify specific stories from my life that can serve as valuable lessons for others and help them navigate life's challenges?

4. What are my aspirations for my children and their descendants, and what blessings do I want to impart upon them?

5. How do I envision my legacy, and what do I want to be remembered for by my loved ones?

6. Are there any family traditions, cultural values, or customs that I want to preserve and pass on to future generations? Why are these traditions important to me?

7. Have there been influential role models or individuals who have shaped my ethical and moral values? How have they influenced my beliefs and principles?

8. What advice or guidance do I wish I had received earlier in life, and how can I provide that wisdom to my descendants to help them in their life journeys?

9. How have personal growth experiences and transformative moments shaped my ethical perspective?

10. What spiritual or philosophical beliefs have been central to my life, and how can I share these beliefs to inspire and guide my family members?

11. What do you want to be remembered for?

12. How did you make people feel?

Your legacy is the imprint that you leave on the earth that transcends long after you are gone.

Life is what you create of it and your Ethical Will is an opportunity to create something that will say to the world, "This is who I am. All of these moments are the fruit of my labour and my story will be continue right here for everyone else to learn from.

Sample Ethical Will

To My Beloved Family,

Life has been a journey filled with valuable lessons, and I want to share some of those with you. Kindness is a powerful force; practice it daily. Family is your anchor; cherish and support each other. Embrace challenges, for they lead to growth. Never stop learning; curiosity is your greatest ally. Our world thrives on diversity; seek to understand. Forgiveness liberates; let go of grudges.

Gratitude brings happiness; count your blessings. Leave a positive mark; your legacy is love and goodness. Balance work and life; find time for joy. Love unconditionally; it's the most precious gift. Embrace life fully, live with purpose, and carry these values with you. My love for all of you is infinite.

With love,

[Your Name]

My Ethical Will

Signature: _____ Date: _____

Epilogue

In these pages, you've had the space to reflect on your life's richness, share your stories, and express your unique wishes. I hope that it has encouraged you to dream big for your final celebration, ensuring it's as full of wonder, joy, and love as the life you've led.

As you finish The Last Hurrah, may it leave you inspired to craft a last hurrah that truly echoes your journey through life. May your final act be a glorious tribute to your passions, your values, and your path.

Remember, this celebration is the biggest gift that you can give to yourself and those who've journeyed with you—a chance to honor, reflect, and rejoice in the life you've lived.

May your last hurrah be as magnificent as your one wild and amazing life.

"Every man's life ends the same way. It is only the details of how he lived and how he died that distinguish one man from another."

Ernest Hemingway

Acknowledgments

This book, a labor of love and reflection, has been nurtured by many who have touched my life, both directly and indirectly.

To my children, Sean, Cody, and Jennifer, whose encouragement and unwavering support (two on Earth and one in spirit) have been my guiding stars. Your shared life experience of losing your father without a book like this as a guide was instrumental in planting the seed and the transformation of this book. Thank you Jennifer for suggesting to me to have a plan of my own. This was essential in reshaping my myriad thoughts into the narrative of The Last Hurrah.

To my cherished granddaughter, Frankie, your fresh, joyful spirit and profound influence on my life are the legacy behind every word of this book.

To my parents, Jack (92) and Maureen (86). It's about time to plan your last hurrah ! You not having a plan was a huge part of the reason why I wrote this book—this one is for you.

I am deeply thankful to Malia Johnson, the spirited and wise 90-year-old woman I met in a Starbucks in Kihei, Hawaii. Your zest for life and meticulous approach to celebrating it became the catalyst for this book. You are a living reminder of the beauty of embracing life's final chapter with grace and intention. Keep on dancing!

Special thanks to Jess Lomas for her keen eye, her editorial acumen, encouragement and support and to Marisa Doolan for her feedback and comments.

A special acknowledgment to my family, friends, and the numerous souls I've encountered on my journey.

Each of you has enriched my understanding and perspective, weaving into the tapestry of this book.

The forest and nature, my greatest teachers, deserve a profound acknowledgment. In the quiet whispers of the trees and the resilient cycle of the seasons, I have learned the most enduring lessons about life, death, and renewal. The natural world has shown me the beauty of letting go, the promise of rebirth, and the importance of being present in each moment.

I also extend my appreciation to the authors, philosophers, and especially the poets and artists whose works have provided wisdom and solace, shaping my comprehension of life and our final farewells. The many teachers and mentors that I have had along the way.

And to you, the reader, for joining me on this journey—may this book be a beacon, guiding you towards a celebration that truly resonates with the depth and joy of your life.

Mary Ann

Resources

Aging with Dignity   agingwithdignity.org

Five Wishes   fivewishes.org

Advance Care Planning in Canada
advancecareplanning.ca

Dying with Dignity Canada
dyingwithdignity.ca

Free downloadable worksheets on end-of-life care from The National Center on Aging (United States) nia.nih.gov

Epitaphs

Source Reader's Digest, "Funny Last Words." Available at https://www.rd.com/list/funny-last-words. Originally published in January 2023, Author: Sarah Vincent.

Urns

Hagan, Dave. Artful Ashes: A DIY Guide to Creating Beautiful Memorial Urns.

Katz, R. The Memorial Urn: Understanding the Healing Process.

Baines, Barry K., M.D. Writing an Ethical Will: A Step-by-Step Guide to Living Legacies.

We're at the end, a legacy cast,

A symphony that's been grand and vast.

As the curtain falls, and the stars applaud,

My greatest gift to you — is my Last Hurrah.

Mary Ann Burrows

Directory for My Loved Ones

Dear _____,
These pages hold more than instructions. They hold a piece of my spirit, a map of my final wishes, and a reflection of the life I've cherished. This is My Last Hurrah — a celebration of me. May this guide bring you comfort, clarity, and a smile, knowing that every word was penned with love and a touch of my signature style.

My Self-Authored Obituary	Pages	59-61
My Guest List	Page	71
My Self-Authored Eulogy	Page	93
My Last Hurrah Party Plan	Page.	102-105
My Farewell Message	Page	113
My Personal Notes & Letters	Page	116
My Important Documents	Pages	125-134
My End of Life Care	Page	143
My Burial Plan	Pages	147-158
My Epitaph	Page	166
My Final Outfit	Page	173
My Ethical Will	Page	183

Other Books by Mary Ann Burrows

Oh, Monkey!, Friesen Press (2019)

Gator on My Back, Friesen Press (2020)

Maisel, E. (2021), Feeling Your Way into Creativity. In The Creativity Workbook Coaches and Creatives (Chapter 23, pp. 72-76). Routledge.

Monk, L., & Maisel, E. (2021). Expressing Feelings in the Virtual Journaling Group. Transformational Journaling Coaches, Therapists, and Clients (Chapter 42, pp. 267-272). Routledge.

Maisel, E., & Monk, L. (Eds.). (2022). The Forest Journal. In The Great Book of Journaling (pp. 119-125). Mango Media.

One Earth, Natural Narratives Publishing (2024)

Made in United States
Troutdale, OR
04/30/2024

19560396R00116